Home Remedies Toolkit

Your one stop guide to natural remedies

Lauren Gamble

Table of Contents

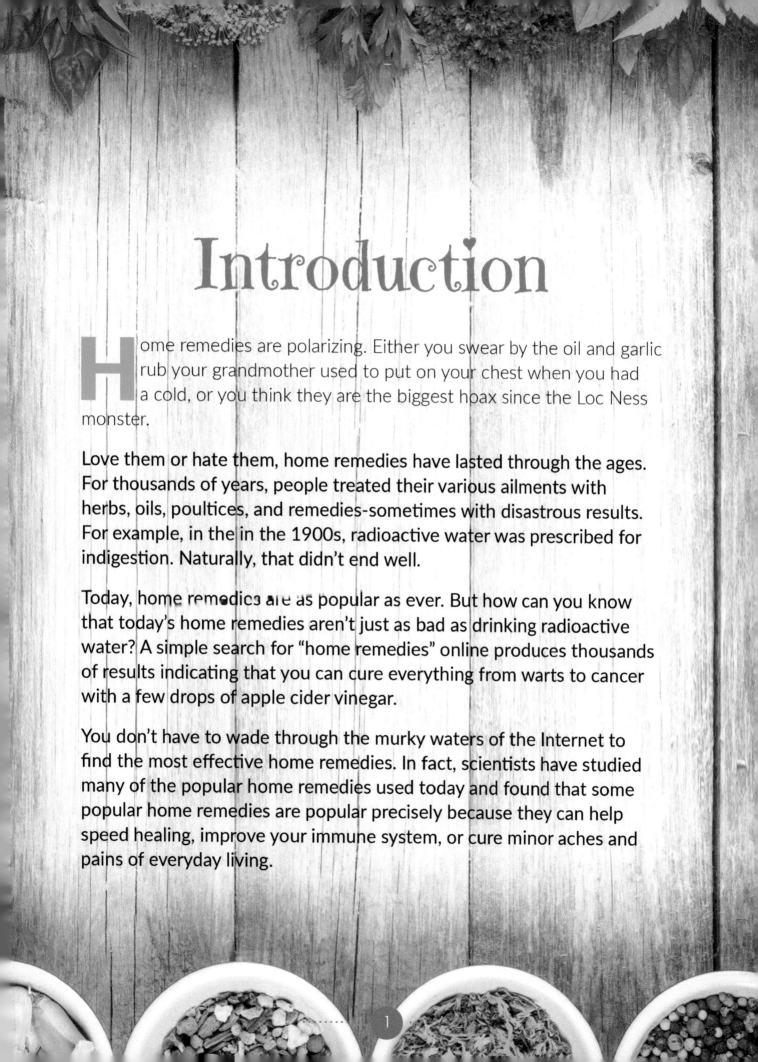

Introduction

Home remedies are polarizing. Either you swear by the oil and garlic rub your grandmother used to put on your chest when you had a cold, or you think they are the biggest hoax since the Loc Ness monster.

Love them or hate them, home remedies have lasted through the ages. For thousands of years, people treated their various ailments with herbs, oils, poultices, and remedies-sometimes with disastrous results. For example, in the in the 1900s, radioactive water was prescribed for indigestion. Naturally, that didn't end well.

Today, home remedies are as popular as ever. But how can you know that today's home remedies aren't just as bad as drinking radioactive water? A simple search for "home remedies" online produces thousands of results indicating that you can cure everything from warts to cancer with a few drops of apple cider vinegar.

You don't have to wade through the murky waters of the Internet to find the most effective home remedies. In fact, scientists have studied many of the popular home remedies used today and found that some popular home remedies are popular precisely because they can help speed healing, improve your immune system, or cure minor aches and pains of everyday living.

If you aren't quite sick enough to visit a doctor but you are feeling slightly under-the-weather, these home remedies are for you.

The home remedies in this guide are backed by scientific evidence supporting the use of that particular substance for the ailments listed in this book. You won't have to worry about trying worthless cures or wasting money on ineffective remedies, as these studies show these home remedies can relieve the symptoms listed in this book.

We hope you use this book as a handy guide to curing the everyday aches and pains that affect your family. In this book you'll find an overview to the studies conducted on each ingredient and what health conditions each ingredient can be used to treat. We've also included a handy quick-use guide that you can use to easily find a home remedy that will treat many common minor health conditions.

Visit the bibliography at the end of the book to find the specific studies referenced in this book for each health condition. A handy number reference for each study is included to make it even easier to locate a specific study.

PLEASE NOTE:

These home remedies are designed to treat minor health conditions. Any serious condition, including but not limited to, high temperatures, illnesses that last longer than a week, and infections that worsen over a period of a few days, should be treated by a doctor. Home remedies are effective in treating minor ailments, but they are not meant to replace prescription medications for serious illnesses.

When in doubt, always visit a qualified health professional.

What You'll Find in this Book

This book is a simple guide to home remedies that work. These home remedies are not only backed by hundreds (and sometimes thousands) of years of use, but they are also backed by scientific evidence and peer-reviewed studies. These studies have shown that for many minor illnesses, home remedies are just as effective as, or only a little less effective, than over-the-counter and prescription remedies for minor health ailments.

In fact, many of the prescription medications used today were derived from natural home remedies and ingredients used hundreds of years ago. In many cases, the prescription versions of a medication use an isolated, strengthened version of the ingredients included in this book. Real medication should always be used to treat serious health problems. We do not advise using home remedies and herbal ingredients to treat conditions worse than the common viruses and health conditions seen everyday.

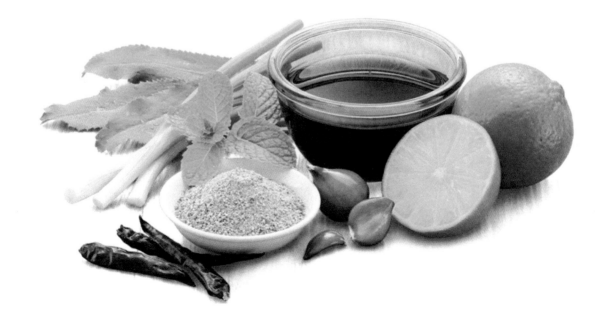

Although we do advise using all tools available in Western medicine for serious health conditions, everyday health problems, like indigestion, colds, muscle pain, and cramps, can be effectively treated at home with these remedies without the need for a doctor's visit or expensive co-pays.

For these everyday conditions, home remedies will provide just enough of a boost to prevent a doctor's visit and help you feel better right at home.

Use this book like a guide to treat everyday illnesses and conditions. Here, you'll find a list of common health conditions and the home remedies that can treat them. For more information on each home remedy, read the section covering the scientific backing for the cures listed in this book.

We hope this book will help you care for your family to the best of your ability using the most natural cures available.

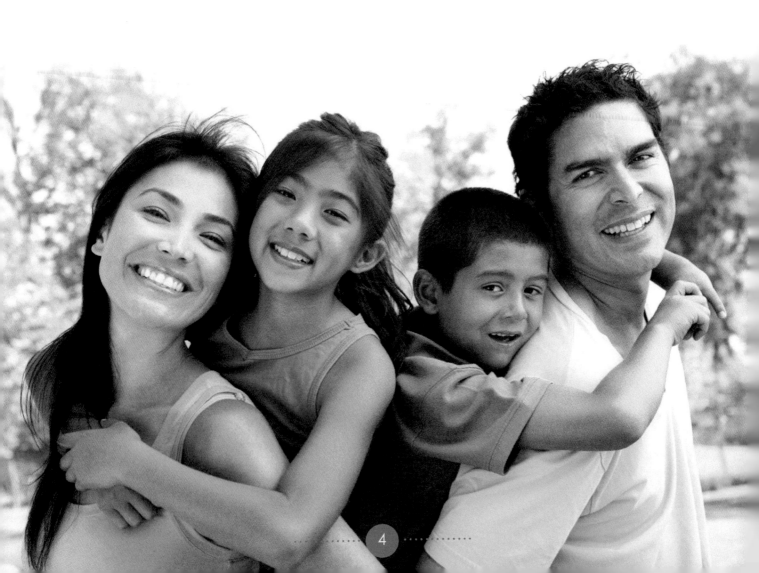

Your Home Remedies Toolkit

If you're just getting started with home remedies, you may be wondering what to add to your home remedies toolkit.

While you can find thousands of questionable uses for various household products (like using candle wax to clean your ears) online, it is much harder to determine where to look for home remedies that actually work.

We've done the research and waded through all the useless remedies to find only the best, most effective ingredients to add to your home remedies toolkit.

Multiple studies have shown that the following ingredients can positively affect the outcome of mild health ailments. Add the following ingredients to your home remedies toolkit and you'll be prepared to face any minor health challenge.

Stocking your home remedies pantry isn't difficult, but if you stock everything at once, it can get expensive. We advise you to pick up one or two of these supplies to have on hand each time you shop.

Store your ingredients in a cool, dry place, such as a pantry. Some of the ingredients may mold if exposed to moisture, so we don't advise storing your toolkit in the bathroom. A shelf in your kitchen or pantry, however, is the perfect place to store these supplies. In addition to the ingredients listed below, keep a supply of bandages, cold packs, heating pads, and iodine for the treatment of minor wounds.

Essentials for the Home Remedies Toolkit

- » Apple cider vinegar
- » Coconut oil
- » Lemon
- » Ginger (raw and powdered)
- » Epsom salt
- » Baking soda
- » Castor oil
- » Olive oil
- » Tea tree oil
- » Garlic
- » Honey
- » Oatmeal

- » Cinnamon
- » Yogurt
- » Aloe vera
- » Peppermint
- » Cranberry
- » Hydrogen peroxide
- » Oil of oregano
- » Green tea
- » Lavender
- » Eucalyptus
- » Elderberry
- » Arnica

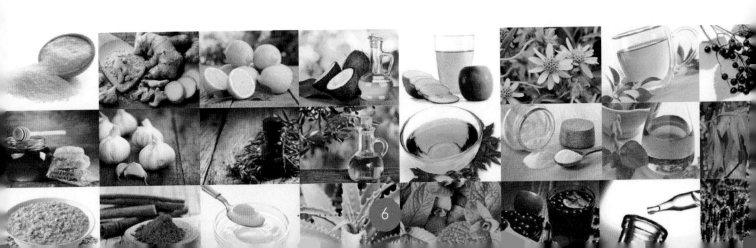

Home Remedies for Common Ailments

Most families are extremely busy. Taking time out of a busy day to visit the doctor for minor aches and pains not only is a major inconvenience, but can also blow the budget.

Home remedies for minor injuries or illnesses (like that pesky common cold!) are attractive, but with thousands of questionable home remedies online it can be a struggle to wade through all that noise and find what actually works.

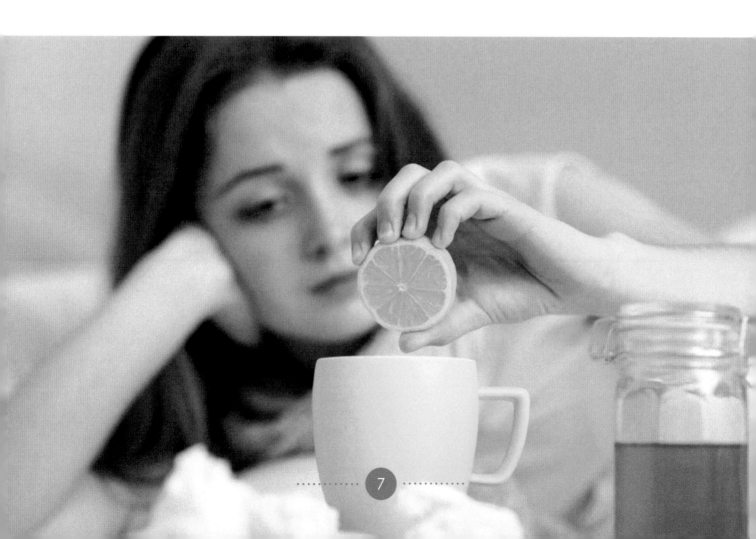

We've eliminated the guesswork and given you only solid, science-backed home remedies that you can use to treat the everyday injuries of your household, including minor colds, smashed fingers, joint pain, and headaches.

This guide is not meant to replace your doctor, but will definitely give you some workable options for those medical issues that are more of an inconvenience than a true health risk.

We've made it easier than ever to find the right remedy for minor health issues by not only using purely science-backed remedies, but we've also create a handy, clickable guide you can use for whatever ailment you're currently facing.

Have an ingrown toenail? Click the condition to be taken to a cheat sheet for treating your sore toe. Have the sniffles? Click the cold chapter for a brief action plan you can use to start feeling better fast.

» Acne	» Dandruff	» Allergies
» Fungal Infections	» Eye injuries	» Bug bites
» Headaches	» Upset stomach	» Itchy skin
» Food Poisoning	» Eczema	» Dermatitis
» Colds and Flu	» Psoriasis	» Ulcers
» Sore Muscles	» Sore throat	» Athlete's foot
» Sore Joints	» Earache	» Eye infections
» Burns	» Warts	» Ringworm
» Sunburn	» Joint pain	» Chilblains
» Ear Infections	» Sprains	» Pink eye
» Dry skin	» Fever blisters	» Molluscum
» Minor wounds	» Bad breath	» Chickenpox
» Edema	» Cramps	» Illness prevention
» Nausea	» Toothache	» Cough
» Constipation	» Gas	

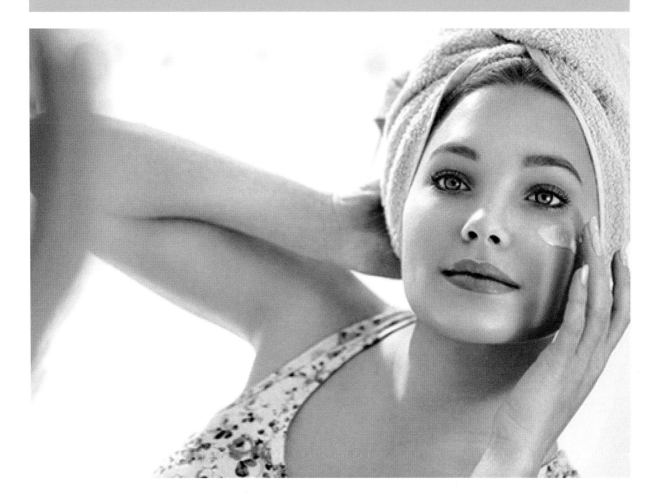

COCONUT OIL

Exchange your regular moisturizer for coconut oil. After washing your face, apply a thin layer of coconut oil in the morning and at night. Use coconut oil twice daily for two months to see full results.

ALOE VERA

After using your regular face cleanser, crush a third of an aloe plant leaf with a fork, blender, or knife. Spread the mixture onto your face and leave it there for 30 minutes. Rinse clean. Apply this mask to your face once or twice a week for cleaner, brighter skin.

TEA TREE OIL

Dilute 5 drops of tea tree oil in a teaspoon of melted coconut oil. Spread the mixture over your face as a daily moisturizer. You can also apply one drop of tea tree oil directly to pimples to speed drying and healing. If you notice your skin starting to peel, discontinue the application of tea tree oil until your skin heals.

FUNGAL NAIL INFECTIONS

TEA TREE OIL

Rub full-strength tea tree oil around and under the infected nail twice daily. The infection should be gone within a few weeks if it is near the surface of the nail.

OIL OF OREGANO

Rub oil of oregano directly onto the affected area three times a day. Get as close to the source of the nail infection as possible. Cover the infected area with an oil-soaked cotton ball and a band aid for a week. The infection should heal within seven to ten days.

HEADACHES

PEPPERMINT

When a headache first starts, dilute 1 drop of peppermint oil into 10 drops of a carrier oil (like coconut oil). Dab the peppermint mixture on each temple. Repeat every 30 minutes until your headache subsides.

FOOD POISONING

HONEY

After a bough of diarrhea or vomiting due to food poisoning, add about a tablespoon of honey to a glass of water. Drink the honey water to stay hydrated and speed the healing process. You can also drink a glass of honey water at the first signs of an upset stomach.

CRANBERRY

Drink cranberry juice at the first sign of food poisoning. Dilute the juice with about 50 percent water to prevent undue digestive stress on the stomach. After you have stopped vomiting for two hours, drink a glass of cranberry juice every few hours to eliminate the rest of the bacteria from your stomach.

EUCALYPTUS

Eucalyptus has powerful antibacterial properties in addition to soothing anti inflammatory properties. Add a drop of eucalyptus oil to water you drink to stay hydrated when dealing with food poisoning. Continue drinking water with eucalyptus oil until symptoms fade. If vomiting last longer than two days, visit a doctor.

COLDS AND FLU

LEMON

At the first sign of a cold (usually a sore throat or sneezing multiple times a day), add the juice of a fresh lemon to a glass of water and drink it. Drink this mixture of lemon water twice daily until cold symptoms subside.

CINNAMON

When cold symptoms hit, add a quarter teaspoon of crushed cinnamon bark to chamomile tea. Drink this cinnamon tea mixture three times a day until symptoms subside.

YOGURT

When you feel a cold coming on, add a cup of live culture yogurt to every meal. Continue eating yogurt daily until symptoms stop.

ELDERBERRY

Take a teaspoon of elderberry syrup three times a day at the first sign of a cold or other viral infection. Continue taking elderberry daily until symptoms subside.

EUCALYPTUS

Rub eucalyptus oil directly onto the chest (using a carrier oil) to loosen phlegm. If you have a sore throat, add a drop of eucalyptus oil to warm water and gargle for 30 seconds. Repeat this gargle mixture until your sore throat is gone.

OIL OF OREGANO

Rub a drop of oregano oil on your chest (with a carrier oil) a few times a day until symptoms have faded.

GREEN TEA

When suffering from a cold, the flu, or another minor illness, rather than just drinking water to stay hydrated, drink green tea instead. Drink several cups of green tea sweetened with honey to soothe cold symptoms and shorten the duration of the illness.

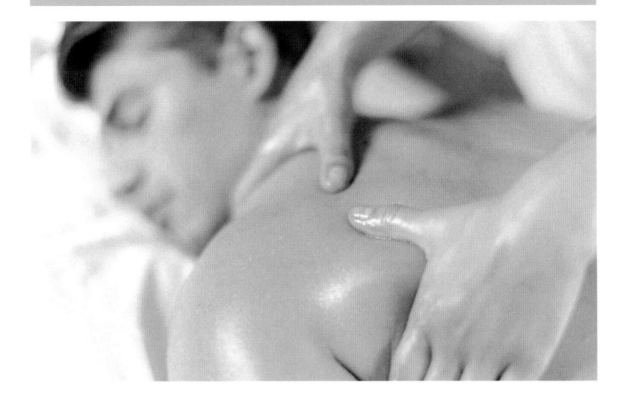

APPLE CIDER VINEGAR

Add two cups of apple cider vinegar to a hot bath and soak for an hour. Repeat once a day until the muscles are no longer sore.

EPSOM SALT

Add 1/2 a cup of Epsom salt to a hot bath. Soak the sore muscle in the tub for an hour to relieve pain and speed healing. Repeat once a day until pain subsides.

CINNAMON

Consume 1/4 teaspoon of salt daily to sooth sore muscles from the inside out. This is particularly helpful when exercising intensely for extended periods.

ARNICA

Rub arnica oil directly onto sore joints twice daily. You can also add a few drops of arnica oil to a warm bath and soak for an hour.

SORE JOINTS

GINGER

Add 1/4 teaspoon of dried or raw ginger to a daily cup of tea to relieve sore joints from the inside out.

EPSOM SALT

Add 1/2 a cup of Epsom salt to a hot bath and soak for an hour to relieve painful, sore joints.

ARNICA

Rub a few drops of arnica oil into stiff, sore joints twice daily, or when joint pain strikes.

BURNS

HONEY

Apply honey directly to a burn as soon as it happens. Cover the wound with gauze to hold the honey in place and speed the healing of the area.

ALOE VERA

Apply the gel from an aloe vera plant directly to new burns. Reapply the aloe as soon as the burn soaks up the aloe (which will vary depending on how severe the burn is). Repeat the application of aloe to the burn for two to three days or until all pain from the burn is gone.

APPLE CIDER VINEGAR

For large burns, add 3 cups of apple cider vinegar to a lukewarm bath. Soak the burn in the vinegar bath until pain is gone.

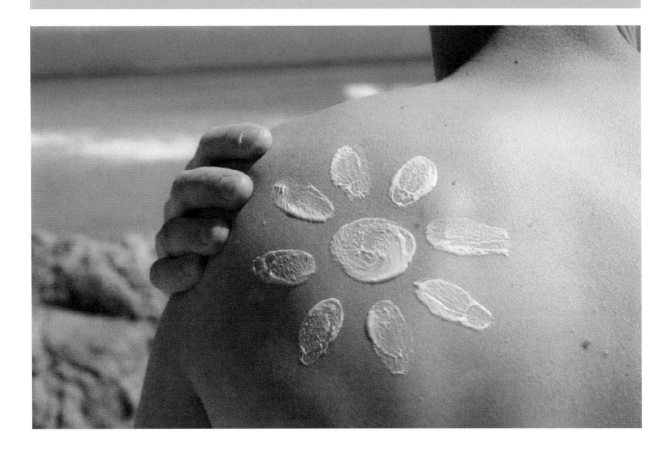

OATMEAL

Make a paste of oatmeal and water. Apply the paste to sunburned skin. Cover the burn with gauze. Leave the oatmeal poultice in place for at least four hours. You can mix this remedy with other sunburn home remedies.

ALOE VERA

Cut a live aloe leaf and split it in half, exposing the sticky center. Rub the sticky aloe gel directly on the sunburn. Re-apply when the skin absorbs the aloe gel. Continue to apple aloe gel until pain is gone.

APPLE CIDER VINEGAR

Mix one tablespoon of apple cider vinegar with one tablespoon of rubbing alcohol. Use an eyedropper to place four drops of the mixture inside the ear canal. Tip your head so the vinegar reaches inside the ear, then tip it the other way to drain the ear. Repeat three to four times a day until pain is gone.

TEA TREE OIL/GARLIC

Crush a piece of garlic and place it in 1/4 a cup of warm tea tree oil. Let the garlic steep in the oil for a hour. Use an eyedropper to drop a few drops of the oil mixture into the infected ear. Wait two hours, then add a few more drops if the pain is still there. Repeat the application every two hours until pain is gone.

MINOR WOUNDS

HONEY

Apply honey directly to the wound after cleaning just as you would apply an antibacterial ointment. Use gauze or a bandage to keep the wound clean until it heals.

ALOE VERA

Once wounds start to heal, rub the gel side of an aloe plant leaf on the wounded area to speed healing and reduce the appearance of scars.

CHAMOMILE

For larger wounds, like abrasions and scrapes, brew chamomile tea and allow the tea to steep for one hour. Soak a rag or gauze in the chamomile tea and wring out most of the liquid. Place the chamomile rag directly over the wound to reduce inflammation and speed the healing process. If the wound is actively bleeding, don't use this method.

ARNICA

Add a drop of arnica oil to scrapes, cuts, and minor wounds to reduce pain in the area. When the wound starts to heal, you can rub arnica oil directly onto the skin for further pain relief.

LAVENDER

Add a few drops of lavender to bandages before applying them over a wound.

APPLE CIDER VINEGAR

Soak a rag or strip of gauze in apple cider vinegar. Ring out the excess and drape over the wounded area. This works best for bruises, scrapes, abrasions, burns, and larger injuries.

NAUSEA

GINGER/PEPPERMINT/CINNAMON

At the first sign of upset stomach, add 1/8 of a teaspoon of raw or powdered ginger and 1/8 a teaspoon of cinnamon o peppermint or chamomile tea. Drink one to three cups of tea daily until symptoms subside. If you start vomiting, wait one hour after vomiting before drinking this mixture.

HEARTBURN

BAKING SODA

Mix 1/2 a teaspoon of baking soda into 4 ounces of water and drink at the first sign of heartburn. Repeat the dosage every two hours until heartburn is gone.

CASTOR OIL

When constipated, make a castor oil pack to relieve constipation.

You will need plastic wrap, a hot water bottle, a large piece of flannel, and an old towel.

Fold the flannel into quarters, making sure it is still as large as your stomach. Soak the flannel in the castor oil. Lie down with your feet propped up.

Place the soaked flannel on your stomach. Cover the flannel with plastic wrap. Place a heated hot water bottle over the plastic wrap.

Place the towel over the water bottle. Remain in that position for an hour.

Repeat this process once a day until your constipation symptoms are gone.

DANDRUFF

TEA TREE OIL

Add 20 drops of tea tree oil to your regular shampoo or conditioner. Wash hair as normal. Additionally, you can add 20 drops of tea tree oil to 1/4 a cup of olive oil and rub directly into your scalp once a day. Continue this treatment until your dandruff is gone.

OIL OF OREGANO

Oregano is a powerful anti fungal agent. If your dandruff is caused by fungus, rub the affected area with oregano oil right after you shower or at night before bed. Let the oil soak into the skin overnight. Within a few days, your dandruff should lessen.

HONEY

Once a week, rub a few tablespoons of honey directly into your scalp. Leave the honey on your head for 30 minutes before rinsing. If necessary, you can increase this treatment to twice a week, or even daily.

OATMEAL

If tea tree oil and honey aren't solving your dandruff problem, try colloidal oatmeal. Apply colloidal oatmeal directly to your scalp once a day and leave in for an hour before rinsing out. Symptoms should start to subside in just a few days.

BAD BREATH

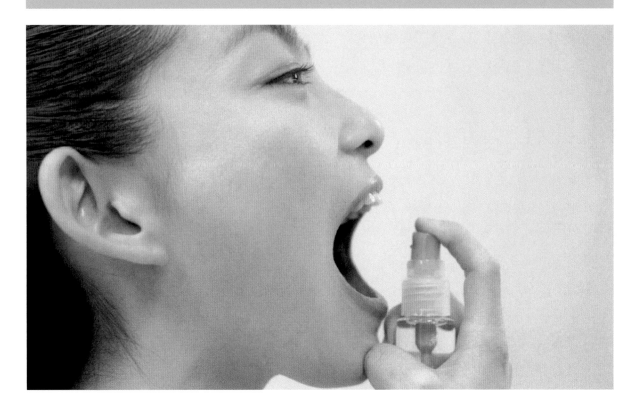

CRANBERRY

Drink cranberry juice daily to reduce halitosis and kill mouth bacteria.

PEPPERMINT

Add a drop of real peppermint essential oil to your mouthwash each morning and night to kill mouth bacteria and discourage plaque from sticking to your teeth and gums.

EUCALYPTUS

After each meal, add a drop of eucalyptus oil to a glass of water and gargle for 30 seconds. This will coat your mouth and teeth with bacteria-fighting compounds that prevent the buildup of bad breath-causing bacteria in your mouth.

GREEN TEA

Green tea contains anti-bacterial compounds that prevent the buildup of plaque in the mouth. Drinking green tea will help keep your mouth clean and your breath fresh.

HYDROGEN PEROXIDE

Rinse your mouth once a day with hydrogen peroxide. Not only will this slightly whiten your teeth, it also discourages the buildup of bacteria in your mouth which can lead to bad bread and cavities.

MENSTRUAL CRAMPS

CHAMOMILE

Drink one to three cups of chamomile tea the week before your period when cramps are most likely to hit. Continue drinking chamomile tea until your period ends.

Red raspberry leaf:

HONEY

Dilute honey with a 50 percent honey and 50 percent saline solution. Apply the mixture inside the infected eye and around the eyelid. Repeat every two hours until pink eye is gone.

TOOTHACHE

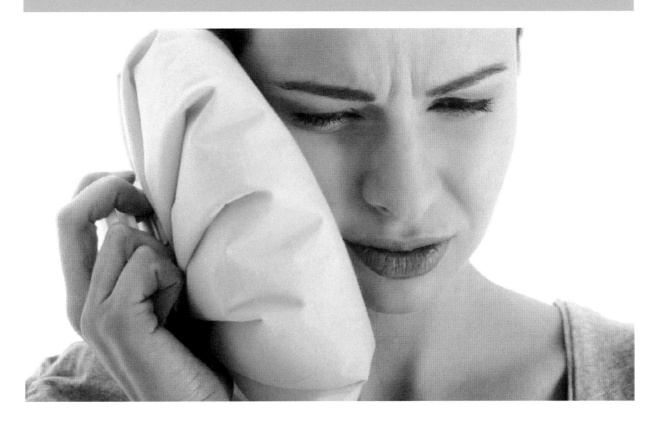

CLOVE

Apply one drop of undiluted clove oil to a painful tooth. Clove will temporarily relieve the pain while also killing some of the bacteria that might be making the tooth sore. Clove should never replace a dentist, but it can be used to soothe tooth pain until a dental appointment is set.

PEPPERMINT/HONEY

When you're feeling gassy, drink one cup of peppermint tea every two hours until symptoms subside.

GINGER/CHAMOMILE/HONEY

Add 1/4 of a teaspoon of powdered or raw ginger to a cup of chamomile tea and drink every two hours until the bloated, gassy feeling fades. Sweeten your tea with honey for even bigger benefits.

BUG BITES

TEA TREE OIL

Apply one drop of tea tree oil to bug bites to kill bacteria and speed the healing of the bite. You can use tea tree oil in conjunction with other bug bite remedies.

OATMEAL

Apply colloidal oatmeal to mosquito bites, flea bites, and other minor bug bites. The swelling, redness, and pain should subside within hours.

LAVENDER

Apply a drop of lavender oil to bug bites to speed healing, prevent infection, and take away itchiness.

DERMATITIS

OATMEAL

Apply colloidal oatmeal to red, itchy skin. Apply the oatmeal twice daily until the redness fades. You can use oatmeal in conjunction with other remedies.

HONEY

Apply honey directly to the irritated area. Let the honey sit for about 30 minutes before washing off. You can use honey in conjunction with other remedies.

COCONUT OIL

Moisturize the itchy skin with coconut oil. Rub coconut oil into the skin until it is absorbed by the skin. You can moisturize the area with coconut oil twice a day until the rash is gone. You can use coconut oil in conjunction with other remedies.

CHAMOMILE

Brew chamomile tea and soak a gauze pad or rag in the tea. Apply the tea-soaked rag to the irritated area and leave in place for 20 to 30 minutes. This will sooth the area, relieve itching, and speed healing. Repeat daily until the dermatitis is gone.

ULCERS

HONEY

If you suspect an ulcer, eat a teaspoon or two of honey each day (it can be taken with food) to encourage your body to quickly heal the problem.

CHAMOMILE

Drink a cup of chamomile tea every day until symptoms subside. The chamomile provides a soothing, anti inflammatory effect on your stomach, relieving pain from ulcers and speeding healing.

HONEY

Apply honey directly to the infected foot. use gauze to wrap the infected area and keep the honey in place.

OATMEAL

If honey isn't working, try applying colloidal oatmeal to the infected area. Apply three times a day until the symptoms are gone.

APPLE CIDER VINEGAR

Soak the infected foot in a solution of 50 percent apple cider vinegar and 50 percent water. Soak your foot for 30 minutes a day until the symptoms are gone. You can use the apple cider vinegar remedy in conjunction with others.

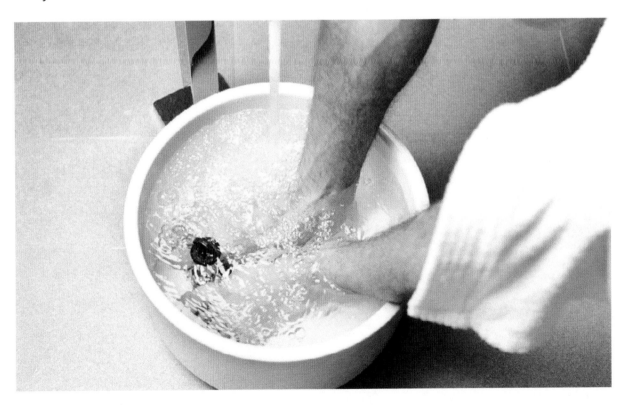

TEA TREE OIL

Rub a few drops of tea tree oil into the affected area. Repeat twice a day until the infection is gone.

LAVENDER

Rub lavender oil into the affected area twice a day until the infection is gone.

OIL OF OREGANO

Rub a few drops of oregano oil into your feet until the oil is absorbed. Repeat twice a day until the infection is gone.

RINGWORM

TEA TREE OIL

Apply a drop of tea tree oil to ringworm spots. Apply the oil four times a day until the infection is gone.

HONEY

Apply honey over the ringworm marks once a day. Repeat until the ringworm is gone. You can use both honey and tea tree treatments at the same time.

EYE INJURIES

HONEY

Apply honey directly to eye injuries including abrasions, minor cuts, and bruises. Honey is healing for the eye condition but also gentle enough to not damage the eye or cause any more pain.

YOGURT

Eat yogurt daily to improve your digestive health.

Peppermint: Drink peppermint tea a few times a week to boost digestive health.

ECZEMA

CHAMOMILE

Soak a rag in lukewarm chamomile tea. Squeeze out the excess and use it to dab areas affected by eczema. Do this twice a day while flare-ups are present.

PSORIASIS

OATMEAL

Apply colloidal oatmeal to affected skin once a day until symptoms subside.

ALLERGIES

YOGURT

Eat yogurt daily during allergy season to lessen the severity of your allergies.

TEA TREE OIL

If you have an allergic reaction to a chemical, bug bite, food, or other substance, drop a few drops of tea tree oil into a carrier oil (like coconut oil) and rub it on the affected area. Tea tree oil can help reduce swelling and prevent infections.

HONEY

Apply honey directly to the blister three times a day. Repeat until the blister is gone (which should be three days or less).

WARTS

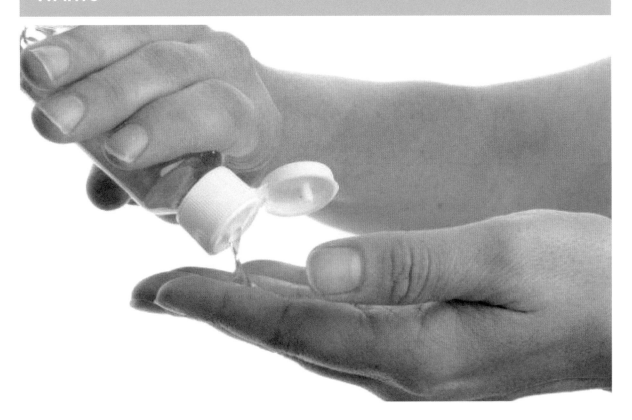

TEA TREE OIL

 Add a few drops of tea tree oil to a wart and cover tightly with a bandage. Every four hours, add a few more drops of oil to a new bandage and recover the wound. Within a few days, the wart should die.

OIL OF OREGANO

Add a few drops of oregano oil to a cotton ball. Place the oil-soaked ball on the wart and cover with a bandage. Leave the bandage in place for a week, adding more oil each day. After a week, the wart should be gone.

CASTOR OIL

Make a castor oil pack to relieve joint pain on the spot. You will need plastic wrap, a hot water bottle, a large piece of flannel, and an old towel.

Fold the flannel into quarters, making sure it is still as large as whatever joint is currently sore. Soak the flannel in the castor oil. Lie down with your feet propped up.

Place the soaked flannel on the sore joint. Cover the flannel with plastic wrap. Place a heated hot water bottle over the plastic wrap.

Place the towel over the water bottle. Keep the castor oil pack in place until the pain is reduced or gone.

GINGER

Take 1/4 teaspoon of raw or powdered ginger daily to relieve chronic joint pain.

SPRAINS

CASTOR OIL/CLOVES

Make a castor oil pack to relieve sprains. You will need plastic wrap, a hot water bottle, a large piece of flannel, and an old towel.

Fold the flannel into quarters, making sure it is still as large as whatever joint is currently sore. Add 10 drops of clove essential oil to your castor oil. Soak the flannel in the castor oil. Lie down with your feet propped up.

Place the soaked flannel on the sprain. Cover the flannel with plastic wrap. Place a heated hot water bottle over the plastic wrap.

Place the towel over the water bottle. Keep the castor oil pack in place until the pain is reduced or gone.

CHAMOMILE

Add chamomile leaves to a warm bath and soak in the mixture until the pain of the sprain is lessened.

ARNICA

Add a few drops of arnica oil to a foot bath or bath tub. Soak the affected area in the warm bath for an hour. Repeat daily until the pain is gone.

SORE THROAT

SALT

Add a teaspoon of salt to a cup of warm water. Gargle with the salt mixture for a few seconds once an hour until the sore throat is gone.

HONEY

Add honey to ginger, chamomile, or peppermint tea and drink one or more cups daily. Whenever your throat hurts, drink a sip of honey-sweetened tea until the sore throat is gone.

EUCALYPTUS

Add a few drops of eucalyptus oil to a warm glass of water and gargle for 30 seconds. Repeat several times a day until the sore throat is gone.

HEMORRHOIDS

CHAMOMILE

Make a strong tea by steeping chamomile leaves (or tea bags) in a few cups of water for several hours. Once the mixture cools, make a sitz bath by filling a shallow container with the tea (make sure it is large enough to sit in).

Sit in the tub for about an hour to sooth hemorrhoids.

You can also apply chamomile topically to hemorrhoids by mixing coconut oil with the chamomile brew. Apply to the infected area several times a day until the hemorrhoids disappear.

EDEMA

CHAMOMILE

Soak an old rag in chamomile tea. Wring most of the tea out, but leave it damp. Lay the damp rag over the swollen area while keeping it elevated for at least 20 minutes. Repeat several times a day until edema is gone.

You can also drink a daily cup of chamomile tea to reduce swelling from the inside out.

CHILBLAINS

HONEY

Apply honey directly to chilblains after exposure to the cold. Wrap the chilblains in gauze to maximize the healing power of honey.

MOLLUSCUM

OATMEAL

If a child has molluscum, make a paste from oatmeal and water. Apply the paste to the infected area and leave it there for at least an hour. Repeat this treatment daily until molluscum is gone.

LICE

TEA TREE AND LAVENDER OIL

Mix a few drops of tea tree oil and lavender oil. Place on the scalp of the affected person three times a day. Run a lice comb through the hair to remove lice and larva from the scalp. Continue applying the oil to the person's scalp for two days after the last lice is seen in the hair.

OATMEAL

Just like your mother did, if chicken pox strikes, the soothing power of oatmeal comes to the rescue. Make an oatmeal soak in the bathtub or make a paste and apply it directly to chickenpox. Repeat several times a day until itchiness and redness are gone.

ILLNESS PREVENTION

Make a disinfecting spray with:

» 10 drops of lemon essential oil or the juice of 2 lemons

» Hydrogen peroxide

Add oil or juice first and then hydrogen peroxide. Store this mixture in a dark bottle.

You will also need a separate bottle filled with white vinegar. Do not mix the hydrogen peroxide and vinegar as this can create a dangerous acid.

To use the spray, first clean the surface with a rag. Next, spray with the vinegar and let sit for five minutes before wiping away. Then spray with the hydrogen peroxide mixture and let that sit for five minutes before wiping away.

A study from the Virginia Polytechnic Institute and State University found this combo to be highly effective against nearly all household bacteria and viruses.

Use this cleaner as your all purpose cleaner in the kitchen and bathrooms.

Studies show that the following ingredients are effective at preventing illness. If someone in your house is stricken with an illness, give extra doses of these ingredients to everyone else in the house. These ingredients are also helpful to take daily throughout cold and flu season to prevent the spread of illness. Add these ingredients to teas, cook with them, or just take them in the morning like a vitamin.

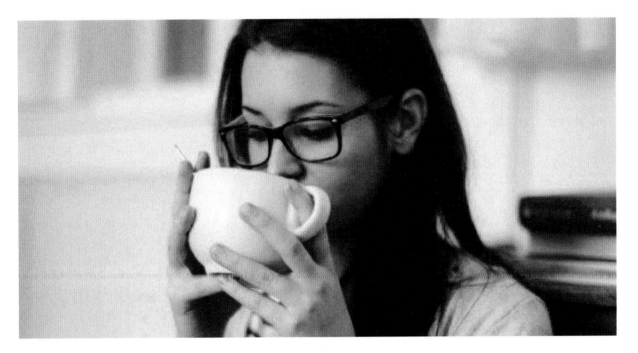

» Lemon

» Garlic

» Yogurt

» Green tea

» Eucalyptus

» Elderberry

EUCALYPTUS

When a cough strikes, rub a few drops of eucalyptus oil directly on the chest to open the nasal passages, loosen phlegm, and make breathing easier. Apply the oil several times a day until symptoms fade.

OIL OF OREGANO

Rub oregano oil directly on the chest (with a carrier oil like coconut oil or olive oil) to relieve coughing and speed healing.

ANXIETY

LAVENDER

Diffuse a few drops of lavender oil in a diffuser to promote a feeling of calm. Rub a drop of lavender oil behind each ear for a long-lasting, anxiety-reducing atmosphere throughout the day.

Science-Backed Remedies

Want to know the science backing the uses of each ingredient in this book? Below, you'll find a complete list of all science-backed uses for common home remedies and how you can use natural ingredients to treat the common illnesses and infections that strike your family. After reading these studies, you might be able to think of additional uses for each ingredient beyond what is listed in this book.

APPLE CIDER VINEGAR

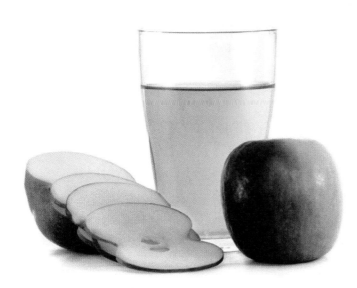

Apple cider vinegar is a popular remedy in the natural health world. It is attributed with numerous health claims including boosting weight loss efforts and killing fungal infections. But with the thousands of health claims behind apple cider vinegar, which are actually backed by science?

According to multiple studies (1, 2, 5), apple cider vinegar is one of the most substantiated home remedies in the world today. The unique blend of acid, fermentation, and fruit make this ancient home remedy useful for many conditions.

Research backs these home remedies using apple cider vinegar:

DISINFECTANT

Apple cider vinegar is mainly made up of acetic acid. This acid is highly deadly to food-borne pathogens. Studies from 2005 (3) and 2003 (4) found that apple cider vinegar is highly toxic to poliovirus 1, bacteriophages, Salmonella montevideo, Escherichia coli and Salmonella typhimurium. Due to these properties, apple cider vinegar is effective for sanitizing, disinfecting, and preventing the spread of foodborne illness. However, it was less effective against non food-related pathogens.

EAR INFECTIONS

A study from 2003 published in The Pediatric Infectious Disease Journal (6) found that apple cider applied topically could speed the healing of minor ear infections, and in particular, swimmer's ear.

SORE MUSCLES

In 2009, a study was published in Anti Aging Medicine (7) that examined the role of acetic acid for the reduction of inflammation and the healing of muscle damage after moderate exercise. It was found that when taken orally, the membrane lipids in acetic acid were able to improve the healing time for muscles after moderate exercise and that total inflammation was reduced.

BURNS

A study from 2000 published in the 14th Forum for Applied Biotechnology, Proceedings (8) found that applying apple cider vinegar to burns sped the healing process. The researchers theorized that the anti-microbial and anti-inflammatory properties in apple cider vinegar decreased the time it took to heal the wounds.

Coconut oil has become ubiquitous in the health scene, but and is prescribed as a remedy for anything from cold sores to weight loss. However, studies suggest that coconut oil is best used for the following health conditions:

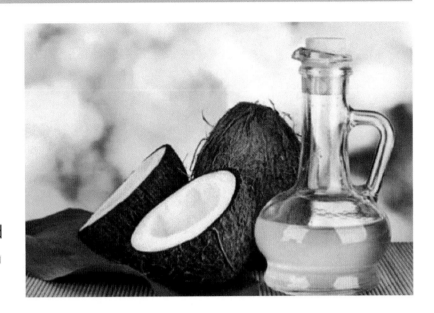

SKIN MOISTURIZER

Coconut oil is a surprisingly effective moisturizer, even though it feels almost rough on the skin. Coconut oil was tested in a study published in Dermatitis in 2004 (1). In the study, coconut oil's moisturizing abilities were pitted against mineral oil. The study authors found that coconut oil was superior to mineral oil and was better able to keep skin hydrated.

WOUND CLEANING

In a 2008 study published in Dermatitis (2), it was found that coconut oil was able to kill 95 percent of staphylococcal colonization on the skin of patients with atopic dermatitis. Other studies have found (3) that coconut oil is powerfully effective at killing bacteria, viruses, and fungi, which makes it effective at preventing wound infections in minor injuries.

ACNE

The antibacterial properties of the lauric acid in coconut oil makes it ideal for fighting acne. A study from 2009 published in the journal Biomaterials (4) found that coconut oil was effective in reducing acne breakouts in study participants.

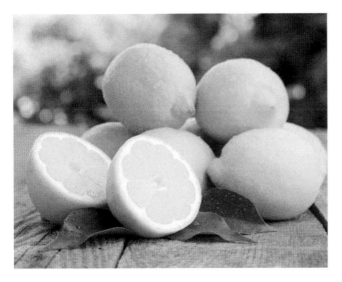

Lemon is a popular home remedy for many conditions- and with good reason. Lemon not only contains high doses of vitamin C, but they also contain B vitamins, copper, iron, potassium, magnesium, and zinc. This powerful mix of nutrients has enabled lemon to be a miracle worker for minor health ailments and injuries.

Science backs the following uses for lemons:

COLD AND FLU

Lemon is antimicrobial and fights viruses, bacteria, mold, fungi, and other pathogens. Lemon is commonly added to natural home cleaning products and laundry detergent for an extra cleaning boost. Due to its antimicrobial properties, lemons can be safely ingested when minor illnesses are present. Lemons will boost the immune system and speed the healing of colds, minor viruses, the flu, and minor bacterial illnesses. (1)

GINGER

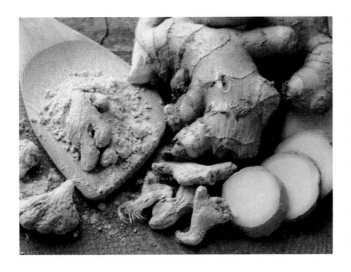

Ginger has been used medicinally in India for thousands of years. However, it was only recently that the practice of using ginger for home remedies was brought to "civilized" countries. Ginger contains powerful compounds that fight inflammation and boost the immune system (1).

How can you use ginger at home? The following ginger home remedies are supported by science:

INFLAMMATION AND SWELLING

While most ginger studies have focused on using ginger internally to find inflammation in swollen, sore joints (1), some evidence also suggests that ginger can help relieve inflammation when used externally as well. A study published in the Journal of Holistic Nursing in 2014 tested ginger's ability to reduce swelling and pain in osteoarthritis patients. At the end of one week of topical application, study participants reported feeling 70 percent satisfied with the pain and swelling reduction.

NAUSEA

Anyone who has ever been pregnant or been around a pregnant woman knows how often ginger is recommended as an anti-nausea treatment. Some women swear by ginger for nausea, while others say it doesn't work.

However, studies do support the use of ginger for nausea, although not for the reason you might expect. According to multiple studies (1), ginger works to relieve nausea by breaking up and expelling intestinal gas.

As for true nausea, a study from 1982 published in The Lancet found that consuming ginger root before a sea voyage was more effective at preventing seasickness than a placebo. A more recent study from 2009 (4) found that women who took ginger supplements in the first trimester of pregnancy reported less nausea and vomiting with no side effects.

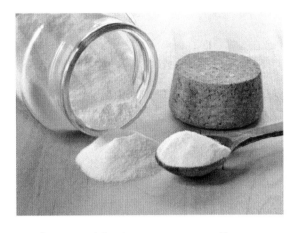

Baking soda (or its scientific name sodium bicarbonate) is yet another ingredient found on almost every home remedy checklist. It has been credited with curing sore throats to healing bladder infections, but not all home remedies for baking soda are effective. In fact, few studies have examined the effectiveness of baking soda used in home remedies.

However, science does support the use of baking soda for this remedy.

HEARTBURN

Baking soda is a base. Most heartburn is caused by the buildup of too much acid in the stomach. A report from Healthline published in 2016 (3) stated that in small doses, baking soda can have a neutralizing effect on heartburn. Many over the counter antiacid tablets contain baking soda.

EPSOM SALT

If you ever had chicken pox or poison ivy as a child, your mother or father probably set you in a tub of Epsom salt to soak. Epsom salt is simply a brand name for magnesium sulfate, which is a mineral compound high in magnesium. Epsom salt has been used for many treatments from fighting fevers to soothing sunburn.

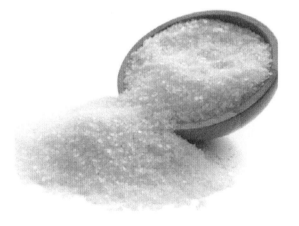

However, studies on Epsom salt are scarce and often have conflicting results.

SORE MUSCLES

One consistent result backs the idea of using Epsom salt to treat muscle pain. A study published in the Journal of Integrative Medicine in 2015 (1) confirmed the results of previous studies. In this study, 24 patients with fibromyalgia sprayed their skin with a solution of water and Epsom salt on their arms and legs twice daily for a month. At the end of the study, the participants reported less daily pain. This suggests that Epsom salt soaks can reduce pain and stiffness in muscles and joints.

CHAMOMILE

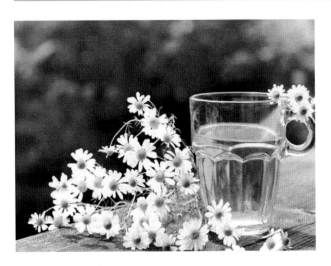

Chamomile is a common herb in every herbalist's toolkit. Not surprisingly, science backs the use of chamomile for several conditions, including:

MENSTRUAL CRAMPS

A study published in the Journal of Agriculture and Chemistry found that drinking chamomile tea increased levels of hippurate in the blood, which is a natural anti-inflammatory and mild pain reliever. This anti-inflammatory response decreases the production of prostaglandin, which causes menstrual cramps. (1)

WOUND HEALING

Chamomile contains properties than when applied externally to wounds, speeds wound drying and encourages new skin to form over the wound faster. (1)

SWELLING

Anti-inflammatory compounds in chamomile work to reduce swelling in sprains, edema, and bloating. (1)

UPSET STOMACH AND ULCERS

Chamomile has soothing, anti-inflammatory properties that counteract an upset stomach. Notably, chamomile has been shown in studies to relieve colic, gas, ulcers, and other stomach irritation (1).

ECZEMA

Topical application of chamomile has been found to be somewhat effective in soothing and relieving eczema (1). Chamomile applied to itchy skin had a soothing effect that reduce itchiness and redness.

HEMORRHOIDS

Studies suggest that chamomile ointment may improve hemorrhoids (1). Tinctures of chamomile can also be used in a sitz bath format. Tincture of Roman chamomile may reduce inflammation associated with hemorrhoids.

CASTOR OIL

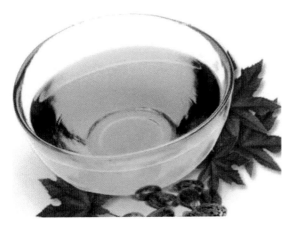

Castor oil has fallen out of favor in the natural home remedies market in recent decades, but your grandparents were likely given a daily dose of castor oil to fight off any impending illnesses. But is there any scientific backing for this mass dosing of WWI and WWI era children? Surprisingly enough, there is some evidence that castor oil can benefit certain minor health conditions.

BACTERIA KILLER

A 2011 study published in the International Journal of Pharmaceutical Sciences and Research (1) found that castor oil was effective in killing gram-positive and gram-negative bacteria. This indicates castor oil can be effective in preventing the spread of bacteria and foodborne illnesses.

ANTI-INFLAMMATORY

In 2000, a study was published in Mediators of Inflammation (2) examining the anti-inflammatory properties of castor oil. The study authors stated that castor oil was as effective as capsaicin (found in cayenne pepper and other spicy foods) at relieving inflammation.

JOINT PAIN

In 2009, a study examined the usefulness of castor oil for relieving arthritis pain (3). The randomized, double-blind, comparative clinical study, study participants were either given 0.9 mL of castor oil in a capsule taken thrice daily or 50 mg of diclofenac sodium. Both groups reported improvement in symptoms after four weeks, but the castor oil group reported no side effects.

CONSTIPATION

A study from 2010 (4) examined the effectiveness of castor oil packs on constipation in elderly study participants. The study authors found that using castor oil packets relieved constipation by making stool easier to pass, relieving symptoms of constipation.

OLIVE OIL

Olive oil has been used in home remedies almost as long as it has existed. The oil contains high levels of vitamin E, antioxidants, and is one of the most beneficial oils for brain health and overall health. You'll see olive oil included in a wide range of home remedies, from moisturizing

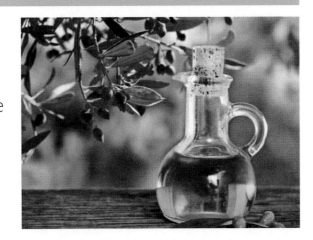

the skin to stimulating hair growth. But which of these home remedies actually provides real results?

Studies have shown that olive oil is an effective home remedy for the following minor health conditions:

HAIR CONDITIONER

A study from 2005 published in the Journal of Cosmetic Science (1) found that while olive oil used in large amounts did cause hair clumping, using a little bit of oil massaged into the hair follicles over time gradually reduced the capillary adhesion of the hair fibers. Basically, this means that the hair and scalp are able to absorb olive oil, which improves the appearance of hair, reduces the damage caused by heating tools, and generally moisturizes the scalp and hair.

OLIVE OIL NOT RECOMMENDED AS A MOISTURIZER

Surprisingly enough, olive oil is not good for the skin. According to a study published in Pediatric Dermatology in 2013 (2), olive oil has a negative effect on the skin's natural barrier against infection. In the study, adult participants applied olive oil to their arms daily for four weeks. The skin's natural barrier against infection and invaders was measured before the four-week application of olive oil and after. The study authors found that not only did the application of olive oil reduce the skin's protective barrier, but that it caused redness of the skin where it was applied, even if the study participants did not have skin problems previous to the study.

Other oils are better suited to topical use as a moisturizer, including coconut oil.

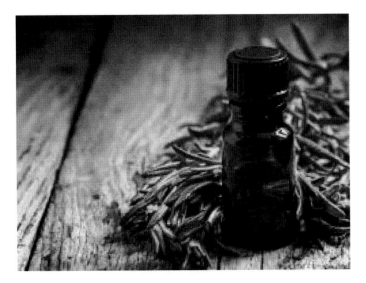

Tea tree oil is a classic and powerful oil used in many home remedies. Sometimes it is called melaleuca oil, and it is effective in several home remedies. Notable remedies are listed below:

ACNE

The home remedy use for tea tree oil that is the most studied and beneficial is in the treatment of acne. Multiple studies have found that tea tree oil is highly effective at reducing acne flare-ups and preventing new pimples from forming. A study from 2007 published in the Indian Journal of Dermatology, Venereology, and Leprology (1) found that a gel containing tea tree oil applied to acne pimples was between three and five times more effective at reducing acne than the placebo gel.

ALLERGIC REACTIONS AND BUG BITES

A study from 2002 published in the British Journal of Dermatology (3) found that tea tree oil was effective in reducing histamine reactions when applied to bug bites, hives, and other inflammation caused by histamines. The study authors found it only took ten minutes before the inflammation was visibly reduced after applying tea tree oil.

FUNGAL INFECTIONS

A review of several studies on tea tree oil (2) found that tea tree oil is highly effective at killing fungus in the lab. The oil is both able to kill fungus and stop it from reproducing. This makes it effective at preventing the spread of fungal infections such as athlete's foot and warts.

FUNGAL NAIL INFECTIONS

Tea tree oil has also been shown to be effective as a treatment for nail fungal infections. In a study from 1999 published in Tropical Medicine and International Health (4) the study authors found that a topical cream containing 2% butenafine hydrochloride and 5% tea tree oil was able to cure fungal nail infections in 80 percent of study participants within 16 weeks. The fungus did not return after the treatment was completed.

LICE

Tea tree oil is an effective treatment for head lice. In a study from 2010 (5), researchers tested three different formulas for killing lice, including a formula containing 10 percent tea tree oil and one percent lavender oil. The oil mixture was applied daily to children with head lice for a period of 15 days. The researchers found that at the end of the study period, nearly 98 percent of the children treated with the lavender and tea tree oil mixture were lice free.

DANDRUFF

Tea tree oil is used often in dandruff shampoos, but only a handful of studies have looked at how effective the oil is on preventing and treating dandruff. In one study from 2002 (6), researchers tested a shampoo containing five percent tea tree oil against a placebo product. The study participants used the shampoo for four weeks. At the end of the trial period, the participant's dandruff level was measured. The group using tea tree oil shampoo had a 41 percent improvement in dandruff symptoms with no side effects.

Garlic is a remedy that has been used to treat minor health issues for thousands of years. Garlic is known for its antibacterial and antiviral properties and is reported to boost the immune system when taken internally. Whether used internally or externally, garlic is one of the safest and most effective home

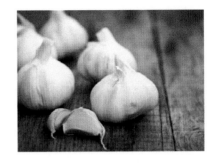

remedy you can use. Raw, fresh garlic contains the biggest health benefits as the compounds in garlic that fight infections slowly fade the longer the root is out of the ground. However, even dried garlic powder can provide some benefits. Studies have found that the following home remedies using garlic are the most effective:

COLD PREVENTION

A review of multiple studies on garlic published by the Avicenna Journal of Phytomedicine in 2014 (1) found that a daily supplement of garlic was able to reduce how many colds study participants caught. Over a 12 week period, study participants consumed a daily supplement of garlic of 2.5 grams per day. During that time, study participants caught an average of 63 percent fewer colds than the control group. Additionally, the garlic takers who did get a cold had their symptoms reduced from an average of 5 days in the placebo group to just over 1.5 days. This reduced the length of symptoms by 70 percent.

HONEY

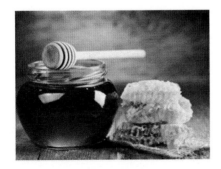

Honey is a powerful remedy that has been used for thousands of years to speed healing. Until recently, most of the information on the benefits of honey came from word-of-mouth and anecdotal sources. However, studies have found that honey is powerfully beneficial in treating many minor health concerns, notably:

WOUND HEALING

Wound healing is one of the top uses for honey(1). Honey was used in WWI as a treatment to prevent wounds from getting infected. Honey was also mixed with cod liver oil to treat burns, boils, ulcers, and other minor injuries. Honey has been extensively studied and it was found that honey could speed the healing of numerous wounds, including:

» Bed sores

» Ulcers

» Cuts

» Abrasions

» Cracked skin

» Burns

» Chilblains

Honey has the unique ability to not only reduce the spread of bacteria (honey is antibacterial), but it can also help stimulate the healing process. Honey was even found to be an effective treatment on open wounds (like cuts) and sped the healing of open wounds without causing any damage to the body.

GASTROINTESTINAL UPSET

Honey was also found to be effective in treating internal gastrointestinal upsets (1). Honey's antibacterial properties make it ideal for treating bacterial-based illnesses, including food poisoning. Honey was also found to be effective in reducing viral infections, such as in the case of rotavirus. Honey was also found to be soothing for individuals with stomach ulcers and sped the healing process for ulcers.

FUNGAL INFECTIONS

Honey is not only antibacterial and antiviral, but it is also anti fungal (1). Honey is able to reduce the spread of fungal infections and has been found to be effective at treating ringworm, athlete's foot, dermatitis, and dandruff.

FEVER BLISTERS

A study published in the Medical Science Monitor in August 2004 found that topical honey was twice as effective as a prescription treatment for fever blisters. Applying the honey to the blister four times a day healed the blister in just three days versus six days when treated with the prescription treatment. Pain was gone after the first day of honey application. (2)

EYE INFECTIONS

Honey is a strange substance because it is detrimental to bacteria, viruses, and fungal infections, but it is extremely gentle on skin and does not cause inflammation or irritation when applied topically. This makes it ideal for treating eye infections. Studies have found (1) that honey can specifically target conjunctivitis, inflammation, and redness in the eyes. Physical damage to the eye also healed faster when honey was applied to the damaged area.

SORE THROAT

Honey has a unique blend of antibacterial and antiviral compounds along with a soothing coating of anti-inflammatory compounds. This makes it ideal in healing a sore throat while soothing the symptoms of a dry, scratchy throat (1).

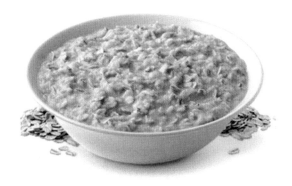

Oatmeal has been used in home remedies about as long as oatmeal has existed. Oatmeal is credited with being one of the healthiest grains to eat, but fewer studies have been conducted on the topical uses of oatmeal.

The Indian Journal of Dermatology, Venereology, and Leprology (1) examined the potential benefits of oatmeal in a clinical review from 2012. This review of multiple studies on oatmeal found the grain to be effective in the treatment of the following conditions:

DRY SKIN

A study on the effectiveness of oatmeal for dry skin (1) found that oatmeal was effective in not only moisturizing the skin within two weeks, but also made the skin barrier stronger.

ATOPIC DERMATITIS

One study examined the potential benefits of oatmeal on atopic dermatitis. For a month, study participants were asked to use a moisturizer using colloidal oatmeal or a moisturizer without oatmeal. The participants who used the oatmeal on their skin had 48 percent improvement in skin health after four weeks and 90 percent improvement after eight weeks (1).

PSORIASIS

Oatmeal has anti-inflammatory properties, which make it ideal in treating psoriasis (1). About three percent of the world's population suffers from psoriasis, which causes dry, scaly patches to appear on the skin. Oatmeal applied to scaly patches of skin reduce inflammation, improve the appearance of the skin, and soothe itching.

VIRAL AND FUNGAL SKIN INFECTIONS

Topical oatmeal has been shown to be effective at killing viral infections. When applied to the skin, oatmeal has been shown to be effective at killing viral infections including molluscum, athlete's foot, dandruff, and chickenpox (1).

SUN PROTECTION

A study in 2003 (2) found that the flavonoids in oats can absorb UV radiation. This makes it an effective protective measure against sunburns and UV damage from the sun. Moisturizers and sunscreens containing oatmeal can help prevent sunburns and UV damage to the skin.

CINNAMON

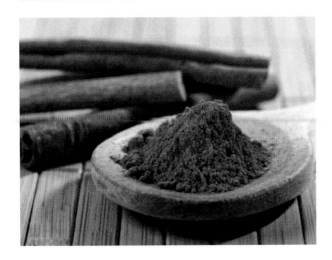

Cinnamon is more than just a spice. Popular home remedies suggest using cinnamon for everything from stopping a cold to removing toxins from the body. However, not every claim about cinnamon is true. The following uses for cinnamon do have scientific backing:

COLDS AND FLU

Cinnamon is able to kill viral, bacterial, and microbial particles. In studies, cinnamon was found to be most effective at killing flu virus molecules, listeria, and e. Coli. (1).

GASTROINTESTINAL UPSET

Because cinnamon is so effective at reducing bacterial and viral infections, it is a powerful remedy against gastrointestinal problems like vomiting, nausea, and diarrhea (1). Studies have found that cinnamon is effective in killing the microbes responsible for causing upset stomach and speeding the healing process.

MUSCLE SORENESS

Cinnamon is not only an infection fighter, but it can also reduce inflammation (2). This makes it ideal for reducing muscle soreness, cell damage, and inflammation in the muscles. In one study on female Iranian athletes, it was found that taking cinnamon powder every day led to significant reduction in muscle pain after six weeks.

TOOTH DECAY

Cinnamon's unique bacteria-fighting properties make it ideal for reducing plaque build up, cavities, and gingivitis (1).

YOGURT

Aside from vague references in yogurt commercials about how yogurt supports digestive health, yogurt has been offered as a treatment for everything from yeast infections to burns. Not all uses of yogurt are backed by scientific evidence. However, there are three clear benefits to yogurt, and one of them is surprising.

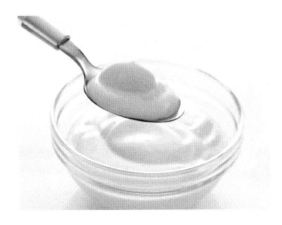

DIGESTION

Not surprisingly, yogurt was found in a review of several studies on yogurt (1) to be effective in improving digestion. Individuals who consumed live-culture yogurt reported fewer gastrointestinal distress, such as fewer upset stomachs and improved digestion overall.

IMMUNE SYSTEM

The same study on yogurt (1) found that daily consumption of live-culture yogurt decreased the instances of colds, flu, and other minor illnesses in everyone who consumed the yogurt. It didn't matter what else the study participants ate, eating more yogurt improved their immune system overall.

ALLERGIES

The most surprising reveal of the study was yogurt's effect on allergies (1). When the blood of the study participants was tested, it was found that those consuming live-culture yogurt had fewer allergens in their system than the non-yogurt group. Additionally, those eating yogurt daily had fewer allergy symptoms like coughing, runny noses, and wheezing.

ALOE VERA

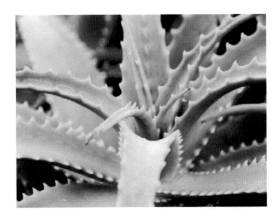

Aloe vera is an amazing desert plant that has healing properties that make it ideal for fighting infections, healing minor wounds, and soothing burned skin. Scientific studies have examined the potential benefits of aloe vera and have found evidence that aloe vera is highly effective in the following uses:

BURNS

Aloe vera is commonly added to skin protection products and after-sun gels for good reason. Aloe vera has a protective effect against UV radiation damage (1). Aloe not only helps heal existing burns, but it also makes it less likely that the skin will be damaged by the sun's radiation in the future.

WOUND CLEANING AND HEALING

Aloe vera can do so much more than soothe burns and sunburn. Compounds in aloe vera (Glucomannan and gibberellin) stimulate the activity of growth hormones, speeding wound healing (1). Collagen production is also boosted when aloe vera is applied to the skin, reducing the appearance of scars. Additionally, aloe vera prevents the spread of infection by acting as an antiseptic agent on wounds. These antiseptic properties work on fungi, bacteria, and viral infections.

ACNE

Anti-inflammatory agents in aloe vera make it a powerful remedy against acne (1). Not only will the anti-inflammatory compounds reduce redness and itching, zinc contained in aloe vera is effective in reducing the bacteria responsible for acne. Compounds in aloe also soften the skin, preventing clogged pores.

PEPPERMINT

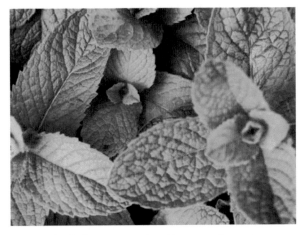

Peppermint is often prescribed to pregnant women in their first trimester to soothe nausea during that time. Anti-nausea is the most well-known application for peppermint, and the most studied. However, peppermint has also been shown to help improve digestion and reduce gassiness, which is beneficial not only throughout pregnancy, but any time of life.

NAUSEA

One study tested the use of peppermint used to relieve nausea in patients with functional dyspepsia (1). In the study, participants were asked to take a peppermint supplement (or a placebo) for one month.

After the month was over, all patients who took peppermint supplements reported less pain, nausea, pressure, and fullness after eating.

GAS

Another study (2) tested peppermint's effectiveness against gas. In this study, study participants either ate a meal containing peppermint essential oil or the meal without peppermint oil. The participants took a breath test that measured gastric emptying four hours after eating. The study authors found that the peppermint oil group had increased gastric emptying, which encourages digestion, relieves gastrointestinal distress faster, and relieves gas.

DENTAL HEALTH

A study from 2013 (4) found that a daily rinse with peppermint significantly improved oral health by killing bacteria and discouraging the spread of bacteria in the mouth. Not only did the peppermint kill bacteria, but it also improved the breath of the study participants previously diagnosed with halitosis.

HEADACHES

A study on peppermint oil tested the use of peppermint oil for headaches (3). In the study, participants were either given peppermint oil to apply topically in conjunction with painkillers or a placebo, or just peppermint oil alone. When study participants had a tension headache, they applied peppermint oil to their foreheads. Within 15 minutes, the study participants reported less pain and tension after applying the peppermint oil.

CRANBERRY

Cranberries are known for their presence on the Thanksgiving table, but little else. However, scientific evidence supports the use of cranberry for the following conditions:

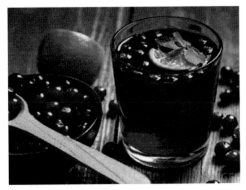

TOOTH DECAY

Cranberry, like many natural foods, has antibacterial compounds. This makes it ideal for keeping your mouth free from bacteria. In addition to simply killing bacteria, cranberries also contain compounds that prevent bacteria from sticking to your teeth, reducing the amount of plaque and cavities (1).

FOOD POISONING

Thanks to the antibacterial properties of cranberry, the fruit is effective at preventing food poisoning (which is great for Thanksgiving). The antibacterial properties in cranberry help prevent the growth of bacteria that cause food poisoning, such as e. Coli. Cranberries (particularly cranberry juice) kill the bacteria before it has a chance to grow and make you sick (2).

HYDROGEN PEROXIDE

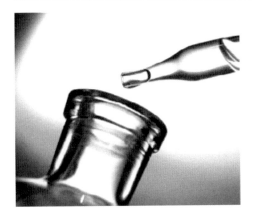

Hydrogen peroxide isn't a miracle cure for all ailments, but it does have two main benefits. Hydrogen peroxide is effective at killing bacteria and viruses, and hydrogen peroxide can also eliminate teeth stains while removing bacteria and plaque from the mouth. Drinking hydrogen peroxide is not recommended.

MOUTHWASH

A study on hydrogen peroxide as a mouth rinse wash was conducted to see if the liquid could improve oral health (1). The study authors found that hydrogen peroxide was beneficial in reducing the amount of plaque and bacteria in the mouth and was also able to lift stains from teeth, boosting the whiteness of the teeth by several shades without causing tooth damage.

HOUSEHOLD CLEANER

Hydrogen peroxide should not be used internally. However, it is effective at killing common viruses and bacteria. In one study (2), study authors found that hydrogen peroxide was effective at killing flu viruses, rhinovirus, e. Coli, and other common bacteria and viruses that can make you sick. Because of its protective properties, hydrogen peroxide is effective at a sanitizing household cleaner.

CLOVE

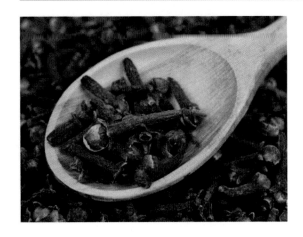

Clove is a wonderfully powerful addition to your home remedies toolkit. It definitely isn't just for seasoning Christmas dishes. Science supports the use of cloves for the following minor health issues:

TOOTHACHE

Studies have found that when applied topically, clove can reduce minor pain (1). This is also true for toothaches. Applying clove oil directly to a sore tooth can dull pain temporarily until a dentist can be seen.

PAIN

A study from 2006 (1) found that clove oil applied to the skin before needle insertion was able to reduce pain significantly in study participants. This indicates that clove applied topically can reduce minor pain.

MOSQUITO REPELLANT

In a study testing several mosquito repellants (2), it was found that only clove oil was effective at repelling all three common species of mosquito for up to four hours.

OIL OF OREGANO

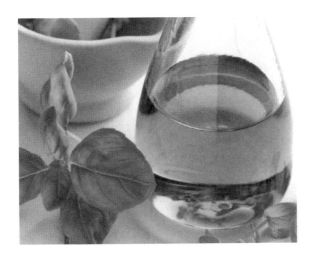

Oregano is a powerful home remedy that can be used for a lot more than simply seasoning Italian dishes. Extracts of oregano are some of the most powerful herbal extracts and the oil extracted from oregano can be used in a multitude of home remedies. Scientific studies back the use of oregano oil for the following conditions:

DANDRUFF

Studies have found that oregano includes powerful anti-viral and anti-fungal properties that are effective in reducing the fungus commonly associated with causing dandruff. This fungus, called Saccharomyces cerevisiae, is killed with the application of oil of oregano, one study published in Phytotherapy Research in 2005 found (3).

COLD AND FLU

An overview of the effectiveness of oil of oregano published in the Journal of Agriculture and Food Chemistry in 2005 found that the oil is effective at killing bacteria and viruses and was particularly effective in killing common flu and cold viruses (1).

COUGH

The Natural Medicines Comprehensive Database lists oregano oil as an effective treatment for coughs (2). This remedy is thanks to the high carvacrol concentration in oregano oil, which encourages the removal of excess phlegm from the lungs and throat.

GREEN TEA

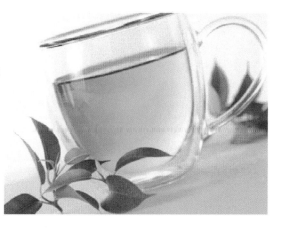

Green tea is often credited with the ability to boost antioxidants in the body and work to prevent cancer, but did you know that green tea also has additional short-term health benefits? Studies on green tea have found that this powerful herb can not only help improve your long-term health, but it can also fight the common cold, the flu, improve your dental health, reduce joint pain, and even boost your immune system. Read on to learn more about the many benefits of drinking green tea.

DENTAL HEALTH

A review on several studies of green tea and dental health (2) have found that green tea is effective at reducing the risk of cavities. Green tea contains compounds that prevents bacteria from sticking to the teeth, similar to how fluoride prevents bacteria from adhering to the teeth.

BAD BREATH

Green tea is also linked with an ability to prevent bad breath. A review on green tea studies published in the Journal of Indian Society of Periodontology in 2012 (2) found that green tea contains polyphenols that kill bacteria in the mouth that causes bad breath. Additionally, green tea powder was show to have deodorant effects, making breath smell even better.

COLDS AND FLU

A review of studies on green tea published in the journal Chinese Medicine in 2010 (1) have found that green tea is effective at shortening the duration of cold and flu viruses. The tea contains antiviral compounds that can work to quickly reduce the number of flu or cold viruses in a person's system and shorten the duration of a cold by several days and lesson symptoms like sneezing, coughing, and runny noses.

JOINT PAIN AND STIFFNESS

A study published in the Journal of Indian Society of Periodontology in 2012 (2) found that when consumed regularly, green tea has anti-inflammatory effects. Study participants suffering from rheumatoid arthritis reported less stiffness and pain in their joints after drinking three to four cups of green tea daily for a period of several months.

IMMUNITY SUPPORT

The 2010 Chinese Medicine review (1) found that when consumed long-term, the antioxidants and antiviral properties in green tea were able to boost the immune system and help prevent the onslaught of common illnesses. The study authors found that study participants who consumed green tea regularly reported getting sick less often than their non tea-drinking peers.

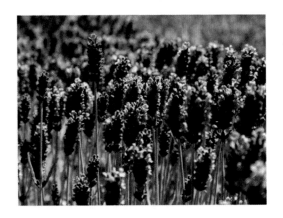

Lavender is more than just a pretty flower and a soothing scent. Although lavender is often used as a flavoring in recipes and a scent for laundry detergent, studies have found that this simple herb can do a whole lot more for your health than most people realize. Lavender can be used as an oil or as an herbal addition to teas, tinctures, and flavoring for food. Read on to see how this simple herb can be used in home remedies to fight minor aches and pains.

FUNGAL INFECTIONS

In 2005, a study published in the Journal of Medical Microbiology (2) found that lavender was an effective remedy against fungal infections. Lavender oil was found to be most effective against fungal strains commonly found on the skin, including warts, dandruff, and athlete's foot.

WOUND HEALING

In 2014, researchers from Celal Bayar University published their findings of a study on the wound healing benefits of lavender oil in Evidence-Based Complementary and Alternative Medicine (3). In this study, the researchers compared the effects of using lavender oil to treat minor cuts in lab rats. The study authors found that wounds dressed with lavender oil healed faster and had less instances of infection than wounds treated using iodine or saline.

ANXIETY

Lavender has been used for hundreds of years to treat minor anxiety and to promote a feeling of calm and wellbeing. However, it was not until recently that researchers began to study just how lavender may affect anxiety. In 2013, Dr. Siegfried Kasper, Prof., MD, from the Medical University of Vienna in Austria reviewed several studies on the effects of lavender for anxiety (4). He found that lavender, taken internally as a capsule supplement was effective at reducing anxiety. In fact, in several clinical trials run by Dr. Kasper, study participants suffering from general anxiety disorder showed reduced symptoms of anxiety after taking lavender supplements within just two weeks.

LICE

A study published in BMC Dermatology in 2010 (5) found that a combination of lavender oil and tea tree oil was an effective remedy against lice. The oils created a suffocating effect that killed the lice and prevented them from breeding.

EUCALYPTUS

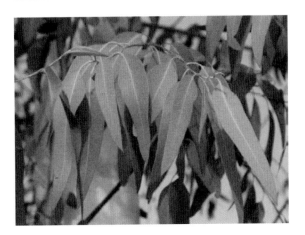

Eucalyptus is another commonly used home remedy for a wide variety of conditions, including dental health, cold and flu prevention, coughs, and sore muscles. But which of these uses are effective? While studies have not found backing for every use listed for eucalyptus online, studies have found evidence supporting the use of eucalyptus= for the following minor health issues.

COLD AND FLU

A study published in the journal BMC Immunology in 2008 (2) uncovered the healing power of eucalyptus oil. Researchers found that eucalyptus has unique properties that make it useful for shortening the duration of colds by boosting the immune system. Compounds in the leaves make it especially useful for sore throats, sinus trouble, and bronchitis. The unique properties of eucalyptus open the nasal passages and encourage the loosening of phlegm in the lungs.

COUGH

The Asian Pacific Journal of Tropical Biomedicine published a study in 2012 (1) highlighting the effectiveness of eucalyptus oil against coughs and bacteria. The plant contains compounds that are highly effective in killing bacteria and viruses. Eucalyptus is particularly effective as an expectorant, loosening phlegm in the lungs and preventing secondary infections like bronchitis.

DENTAL HEALTH

The antibacterial properties of eucalyptus make it particularly effective at reducing plaque build-up on the teeth. The 2012 study (1) found that gargling with eucalyptus could coat the mouth and teeth with an antiseptic called cineole, which can kill bacteria that causes bad breath and reduce plaque build-up on the teeth.

FOOD POISONING

In a study published in 2012 in the Asian Pacific Journal of Tropical Biomedicine (1), researchers found eucalyptus extract effective at killing e. Coli bacteria. This supports the use of eucalyptus oil for food poisoning and other food-borne illnesses.

ELDERBERRY

Elderberry is a curious berry used for hundreds of years as a food, but also as an herbal supplement. Extracts of the berry are often prescribed when a person is suffering from a mild illness, such as a cold or the flu. According to a study published in Phytochemistry in 2009, it was found that during in vitro studies, elderberry was able to kill flu viruses quickly and efficiently. Evidence

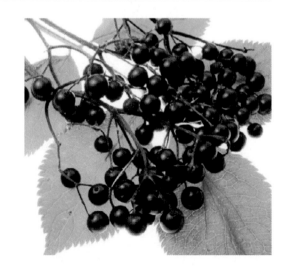

supports the use of elderberry for shortening the duration and severity of minor viruses.

IMMUNE SYSTEM BOOSTER

A study published in 2001 in the journal European Cytokine Network (1) found that elderberry extract was effective not just at killing bacteria and viruses, but also boosting the immune system. Individuals who supplemented with elderberry while sick showed increasing inflammatory cytokine production, which is a marker of a strengthened immune system. Evidence suggests that elderberries can be an effective remedy for fighting off infections and illnesses of all kinds.

ARNICA

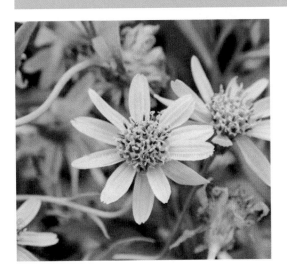

Arnica is a commonly prescribed treatment in the natural health world for conditions such as bruising, joint pain, swelling, sprains, and other mild injuries. Arnica is credited with the ability to act as a mild pain reliever and lesson the length of time pain is experienced. Find out what uses for arnica are supported by scientific evidence below.

PAIN RELIEF

There are few studies on the pain-relieving properties of Arnica extracts, But one study published in Alternative Therapies in Health and Medicine in 2002 examined the use of arnica for pain relief on patients who had just undergone surgery for carpal tunnel. Both homeopathic remedies and ointment containing arnica were applied to the healing area after surgery. After two weeks, the arnica group reported less pain than the group treated without arnica. This suggests that arnica does have pain-relieving properties that can reduce the duration of injuries and pain by several days or weeks, depending on the severity of the injury.

Summary

Home remedies can be a viable replacement for over-the-counter medication when used properly. The home remedies outlined in this guide provide an insider look at which home remedies actually work effectively. There are a million and one different home remedies out there, but the vast majority of them are simply a waste of time and money.

Use this guide to speed the healing of minor injuries and ailments in your family. When you have a minor health issue, pull up your book, click on the appropriate health condition, and apply whatever remedy you happen to have on hand. Most conditions can be treated with several home remedies. It is not recommended to stack remedies, as this could cause other problems like skin irritation. Stick to one remedy at a time, and if the first thing you try doesn't work, you can try something else the next day.

If your condition has not improved within 48 hours, it may be too serious for home remedies. If you don't see any signs of improvement after 48 hours, a visit to a doctor may be warranted. Don't ignore serious medical red flags just because you are treating the condition with a home remedy. Occasionally, even minor health problems require a visit to a doctor.

If anyone in your family is immune-compromised, consult with a doctor before trying any home remedies. Additionally, do not mix home remedies with prescription or over-the-counter medications, as a reaction could occur. Some home remedies may counteract medication you are taking, or may cause similar results, leading to an overdose of a certain ingredient.

If you plan to continuously use a home remedy, consult with your doctor before trying it in case there is a possible interaction with another medication you may be taking. Always err on the side of caution and don't stack medications or multiple home remedies, particularly ones that are internal.

Index

Bibliography

Apple Cider Vinegar

1. Johnston C, PhD, RD and Gaas C BS. Vinegar: Medicinal Uses and Antiglycemic Effect, MedScape General Medicine: 2006.

2. Aykin E, Budak N, Guzel-Seydim Z, Greene A, Seydim A, Functional Properties of Vinegar, Journal of Food Science: 2014.

3. Sengun IY, Karapinar M. Effectiveness of household natural sanitizers in the elimination of Salmonella typhimurium on rocket (Eruca sativa Miller) and spring onion (Allium cepa L.), International Journal of Food Microbiolgy: 2005.

4. Luksik J, Bradley ML, Scott TM, et al. Reduction of poliovirus 1, bacteriophages, Salmonella montevidea, and Escherichia coli 0157:H7 on strawberries by physical and disinfectant washes, Journal of Food Protection. 2003.

5. Rutala WA, Barbee SL, Agular NC, Sobsey MD, Weber DJ, Antimicrobial activity of home disinfectants and natural products against potential human pathogens, Infection Control and Hospital Epidemiology. 2000.

6. Dohar JE., Evolution of management approaches for otitis externa, The Pediatric Infectious Disease Journal. 2003.

7. Sugiyama K, Sakakibara R, Tachimoto H, Kishi M, Kaga T, Tabata I., Effects of acetic acid bacteria supplementation on muscle damage after moderate-intensity exercise, Journal of Anti-Aging Medicine. 2009.

8. Krystynowicz A, Czaja W, Pomorski L, Kolodziejczyk M, Bielecki S, The evaluation of usefulness of microbial cellulose as a wound dressing material.14th Forum for Applied Biotechnology, Proceedings Part 1.

Gent, Belgium: Meded Fac Land-bouwwet-Rijksuniv Gent, 2000.

9. Susan Sumner MD, Vinegar and Hydrogen Peroxide as Disinfectants, Science News: Virginia Polytechnic Institute and State University, 1996.

Coconut Oil

1 Agero AL, Verallo-Rowell VM, A randomized double-blind controlled trial comparing extra virgin coconut oil with mineral oil as a moisturizer for mild to moderate xerosis, Dermatitis. 2004.

2 Verallo-Rowell VM, Dillague KM, Syah-Tjundawan BS, Novel antibacterial and emollient effects of coconut and virgin olive oils in adult atopic dermatitis, Dermatitis. 2008.

3. Kabara J, Swieczkowski D, Conley A, and Truant J, Fatty Acids and Derivatives as Antimicrobial Agents, Antimicrob Agents Chemotherapy. 1972.

4. Yang D, Pornpattananangkul D, Nakatsuji T, Chan M, Carson D, Huang CM, Zhang L, The antimicrobial activity of liposomal lauric acids against Propionibacterium acnes, Biomaterials. 2009.

Lemon

1 Shaik-Dasthagirisaheb YB , Varvara G , Murmura G , Saggini A , Caraffa A , Antinolfi P , Tete' S , Tripodi D , Conti F , Cianchetti E, Toniato E , Rosati M , Speranza, L , Pantalone A , Saggini R , Tei M , Speziali A , Conti P , Theoharides TC , Pandolfi F, Role of vitamins D, E and C in immunity and inflammation, Journal of Biological Regulators and Homeostatic Agents. 2013.

Ginger

1. Benzie IFF, Wachtel-Galor S, Herbal Medicine: Biomolecular and Clinical Aspects, 2011.

2. Tessa Therkleson, PhD, RN, Topical Ginger Treatment With a Compress

or Patch for Osteoarthritis Symptoms, Journal of HOlistic Nursing. 2014.

3. Mowrey D. B, Clayson D. E., Motion sickness, ginger, and psychophysics, Lancet. 1982.

4. Ozgoli G, Goli M, Simbar M., Effects of ginger capsules on pregnancy, nausea, and vomiting. Journal of Alternative Complementary Medicine. 2009.

Baking Soda

1. Mankodi SM, Conforti N, Berkowitz H., Efficacy of baking soda-containing chewing gum in removing natural tooth stain, Compendium of Continuing Education in Dentistry. 2001.

2. Eksp Klin, Evaluation of action, efficacy, and onset dynamics of a single dose of alginates in patients with heartburn and GERD, Gastroenterology. 2009.

3. Cherney K, Marcin J, MD, Can Store-Bought Baking Soda Really Treat Acid Reflux?, Healthline. 2016.

Epsom Salt

1. Engen DJ, McAllister SJ, Whipple MO, Cha SS, Dion LJ, Vincent A, Bauer BA, Wahner-Roedler DL, Effects of transdermal magnesium chloride on quality of life for patients with fibromyalgia: a feasibility study, Journal of Integrative Medicine. 2015.

Castor Oil

1. Kota & Manthri, Antibacterial activity of ricinus communis leaf extract, International Journal of Pharmaceutical Sciences and Research. 2011.

2. Vieira C, Evangelista S, Cirillo R, Lippi A, Maggi CA, Manzini S., Effect of ricinoleic acid in acute and subchronic experimental models of inflammation, Mediators of Inflammation. 2000.

3. B Medhi, K Kishore, U Singh, S D Seth, Castor oil is safe and effective in the treatment of patients with osteoarthritis, Phytotherapy Research. 2009.

4. Arslan Gülşah Gürol, An examination of the effect of castor oil packs on constipation in the elderly, Complementary Therapies in Clinical Practice. 2011.

Olive Oil

1. K. Keis, D. Persaud, Y. K. Kamath, and A. S. Rele, Investigation of penetration abilities of various oils into human hair fibers, Journal of Cosmetic Science. 2005.

2. Danby SG1, AlEnezi T, Sultan A, Lavender T, Chittock J, Brown K, Cork MJ., Effect of olive and sunflower seed oil on the adult skin barrier: implications for neonatal skin care, Pediatric Dermatology. 2012.

Tea Tree Oil

1. Enshaieh S, Jooya A, Siadat AH, Iraji F., The efficacy of 5% topical tea tree oil gel in mild to moderate acne vulgaris: a randomized, double-blind placebo-controlled study, Indian Journal of Dermatology, Venereology and Leprology. 2007.

2. F. Carson, K. A. Hammer,1 and T. V. Riley, Melaleuca alternifolia (Tea Tree) Oil: a Review of Antimicrobial and Other Medicinal Properties, Clinical Microbiology. 2006.

3. Koh KJ, Pearce AL, Marshman G, Finlay-Jones JJ, Hart PH., Tea tree oil reduces histamine-induced skin inflammation, British Journal of Dermatology. 2002.

4. Syed TA, Qureshi ZA, Ali SM, Ahmad S, Ahmad SA., Treatment of toenail onychomycosis with 2% butenafine and 5% Melaleuca alternifolia (tea tree) oil in cream, Tropical Medicine & International Health. 1999.

5. Barker SC, Altman PM. A randomised, assessor blind, parallel group

comparative efficacy trial of three products for the treatment of head lice in children--melaleuca oil and lavender oil, pyrethrins and piperonyl butoxide, and a "suffocation" product, BMC Dermatology. 2010

6. Wu S, Patel KB, Booth LJ, Metcalf JP, Lin HK, Wu W., Protective essential oil attenuates influenza virus infection: An in vitro study in MDCK cells, BCM Complementary and Alternative Medicine. 2010.

7. Satchell AC, Saurajen A, Bell C, Barnetson RS., Treatment of dandruff with 5% tea tree oil shampoo, Journal of the American Academy of Dermatology. 2002.

Honey

1. Eteraf-Oskouei T and Najafi M, Traditional and Modern Uses of Natural Honey in Human Diseases: A Review, Iranian Journal of Basic Medical Sciences. 2013.

2. Al-Waili, Topical honey application vs. acyclovir for the treatment of recurrent herpes simplex lesions, Medical Science Monitor. 2004.

Oatmeal

1. Pazyar N, Yaghoobi R, Kazerouni A, Feily A, Oatmeal in dermatology: A brief review, Indian Journal of Dermatology, Veneerology, and Leprology. 2012.

2. D'Orazio J, Jarrett S, Amaro-Ortiz A, and Scott T, UV Radiation and the Skin, International Journal of Molecular Sciences. 2013.

Garlic

1. Bayan L, Koulivand P, and Gorji A, Garlic: a review of potential therapeutic effects, Avicenna Journal of Phytomedicine. 2014.

Cinnamon

1. Kawatra P and Rajagopalan R, Cinnamon: Mystic powers of a minute

ingredient, Pharmacognosy Research. 2015.

2. Mashhadi NS, Ghiasvand R, Askari G, Feizi A, Hariri M, Darvishi L, Barani A, Taghiyar M, Shiranian A, Hajishafiee M., Influence of Ginger and Cinnamon Intake on Inflammation and Muscle Soreness Endued by Exercise in Iranian Female Athletes, International Journal of Preventive Medicine. 2013.

Hydrogen Peroxide

1. Jhingta P, Bhardwaj A, Sharma D, Kumar N, Bhardwaj V, and Vaid S, Effect of hydrogen peroxide mouthwash as an adjunct to chlorhexidine on stains and plaque, Journal of Indian Society of Periodontology. 2013.

2. Mentel' R, Shirrmakher R, Kevich A, Dreĭzin RS, Shmidt I., Virus inactivation by hydrogen peroxide, Vopr Virusol.1977.

Cranberries

1. Lian PY, Maseko T, Rhee M, Ng K., The antimicrobial effects of cranberry against Staphylococcus aureus, Food Science and Technology International. 2012.

2. Zhang L, Ma J, Pan K, Go VL, Chen J, You WC., Efficacy of cranberry juice on Helicobacter pylori infection: a double-blind, randomized placebo-controlled trial, Helicobacter. 2005.

Peppermint

1. May B, Köhler S, Schneider B., Efficacy and tolerability of a fixed combination of peppermint oil and caraway oil in patients suffering from functional dyspepsia, Alimentary Pharmacology & Therapeutics. 2000.

2. Inamori M, Akiyama T, Akimoto K, Fujita K, Takahashi H, Yoneda M, Abe Y, Kubota K, Saito S, Ueno N, Nakajima A., Early effects of peppermint oil on gastric emptying: a crossover study using a continuous real-time 13C breath test (BreathID system), Journal of Gastroenterology. 2007.

3. Göbel H, Fresenius J, Heinze A, Dworschak M, Soyka D., Effectiveness of Oleum menthae piperitae and paracetamol in therapy of headache of the tension type, Nervenarzt.1996.

4. Haghgoo R and Abbasi F, Evaluation of the use of a peppermint mouth rinse for halitosis by girls studying in Tehran high schools, International Society of Preventive and Community Dentistry. 2013.

Yogurt

1. Van de Water J, Keen C, and Gershwin E, The Influence of Chronic Yogurt Consumption on Immunity, The American Society for Nutritional Sciences. 1999.

Aloe Vera

1. Surjushe A, Vasani R, and Saple DG, Aloe Vera: A Short Review, Indian Journal of Dermatology. 2008.

Clove

1. Trongtokit Y, Rongsriyam Y, Komalamisra N, Apiwathnasorn C., Comparative repellency of 38 essential oils against mosquito bites, Phytotherapy Research. 2005.

2. Alqareer A, Alyahya A, Andersson L., The effect of clove and benzocaine versus placebo as topical anesthetics, Journal of Dentistry. 2006.

Chamomile

1. Wangl Y, Tang H, Nicholson J, Hylands P, Sampson J, and Holmes E, A Metabonomic Strategy for the Detection of the Metabolic Effects of Chamomile (Matricaria recutita L.) Ingestion, Journal of Agriculture and Food Chemistry. 2004.

Oil of Oregano

1. Faleiro L, Miguel G, Gomes S, Costa L, Venâncio F, Teixeira A,

Figueiredo A, Barroso J, and Pedro L, Antibacterial and Antioxidant Activities of Essential Oils Isolated from Thymbra capitata L. (Cav.) and Origanum vulgare L., Journal of Agriculture and Food Chemistry. 2005.

2. Oregano, Natural Medicines Comprehensive Database, Therapeutic Research Faculty. Accessed November 20, 2016.

3. Chami F, Chami N, Bennis S, Bouchikhi T, Remmal A., Oregano and clove essential oils induce surface alteration of Saccharomyces cerevisiae. Phytotherapy Research. 2005.

Green Tea

1. Chacko S, Thambi P, Kuttan R, and Nishigaki I, Beneficial effects of green tea: A literature review, Chinese Medicine. 2010.

2. Chatterjee A, Saluja M, Agarwal G, and Alam M, Green tea: A boon for periodontal and general health, Journal of Indian Society of Periodontology. 2012.

Lavender

1. Kutlu A, Çeçen D, Gürgen S, Sayın O, and Çetin F, A Comparison Study of Growth Factor Expression following Treatment with Transcutaneous Electrical Nerve Stimulation, Saline Solution, Povidone-Iodine, and Lavender Oil in Wounds Healing, Evidence-Based Complementary and Alternative Medicine. 2013.

2. D'Auria FD, Tecca M, Strippoli V, Salvatore G, Battinelli L, Mazzanti G., Antifungal activity of Lavandula angustifolia essential oil against Candida albicans yeast and mycelial form, Medical Mycology. 2005.

3. Stea S, Beraudi A, and De Pasquale D, Essential Oils for Complementary Treatment of Surgical Patients: State of the Art, Evidence-Based Complementary and Alternative Medicine. 2014.

4. Siegfried Kasper, An orally administered lavandula oil preparation (Silexan) for anxiety disorder and related conditions: an evidence based review, International Journal of Psychiatry in Clinical Practice . 2013.

5. Barker SC, Altman PM. A randomised, assessor blind, parallel group comparative efficacy trial of three products for the treatment of head lice in children--melaleuca oil and lavender oil, pyrethrins and piperonyl butoxide, and a "suffocation" product, BMC Dermatology. 2010

Eucalyptus

1. Raho G Bachir and M Benali, Antibacterial activity of the essential oils from the leaves of Eucalyptus globulus against Escherichia coli and Staphylococcus aureus, Asian Pacific Journal of Tropical Biomedicine. 2012.

2. Serafino A, Sinibaldi Vallebona P, Andreola F, Zonfrillo M, Mercuri L, Federici M, Rasi G, Garaci E, and Pierimarchi P. Stimulatory effect of Eucalyptus essential oil on innate cell-mediated immune response, BMC Immunology. 2008.

Elderberry

1. Barak V, Halperin T, Kalickman I, The effect of Sambucol, a black elderberry-based, natural product, on the production of human cytokines: I. Inflammatory cytokines, European Cytokine Network. 2001.

2. Roschek B Jr, Fink RC, McMichael MD, Li D, Alberte RS., Elderberry flavonoids bind to and prevent H1N1 infection in vitro, Phytochemistry. 2009.

Arnica

1. Jeffrey SL, Belcher HJ., Use of Arnica to relieve pain after carpal-tunnel release surgery, Alternative Therapies in Health and Medicine. 2002.

Made in the USA
Middletown, DE
13 December 2019